Dr. Sam Sverdlik's
Uncommon Stories

Humor and hope from patients and doctors

Compiled and edited by Lenora Ucko, PhD

Sverdlik Press Durham, NC

Contents: Page

Foreword

Sam Sverdlik, MD (1916-2014), was the quintessential doctor. Founder of the first Department of Rehabilitation Medicine in a general hospital, he was nationally known as a pioneer in his field. During his forty years as Medical Director, Department of Rehabilitation Medicine, at St. Vincent's Hospital and Medical Center in New York City, he established practices that are current today. He served as an adviser and role model for hospitals starting rehabilitation departments, and influenced students, staff, and colleagues alike. He was a skilled practitioner, sensitive clinician, inspired teacher, and an engaging raconteur. We are fortunate to have, in his own words, important moments of Sam Sverdlik's medical career.

Lenora Ucko, PhD, (1921-   ) has a varied background. A cultural anthropologist, she taught at universities in the United States and Europe. She publishes non-fiction for the general public and scholarly works for professional colleagues. An experienced storyteller, she founded a non-profit organization, StoriesWork, and innovated Interactive Storytelling, a technique using folk stories to help people cope with life's challenges. Dr. Ucko was a visiting scholar at the Bunting Institute of Radcliffe University, received research awards from the American Association for the Advancement of Science and the National Storytellers Network, and lectured at The United Nations Committee on the Family and the UN Commission on the Status of Women.

Lenora Ucko and Sam Sverdlik were distantly related, long time colleagues, and mutual admirers.

1. Introduction

After many years of listening to Dr. Sam Sverdlik (1916-2014) talk about his medical practice, I was inspired to collect his stories and make them publicly available. Though events in these stories take place in the second half of the 20th century, the stories are groundbreaking and relevant today. The stories reveal Sam's unique approach to medicine, his skill training others, his startling success with intractable patients, and his empathy with patients, their relatives and caregivers.

Sam and I began recording his stories after we were both retired and living 400 miles apart – he in Florida and I in North Carolina. By this time (2013), we were hampered by Sam's limited eyesight and reduced manual dexterity, and my inability to travel far from home. A story collection plan had to accommodate these restrictions. It was quite a feat!

We were fortunate that though Sam's memory needed occasional jogging, his thinking was as sharp as ever. And I had become familiar with some 21st century technology. Without a moment to lose, we worked out a plan in which we would use the telephone, a digital recorder, and the computer. We spoke to each other over the telephone. Then with the digital recorder next to my phone, I could record Sam recounting his stories and I finally uploaded them into the computer. This we did throughout the year. Using modern technology, we overcame miles of separation without forfeiting personal interactions.

Once the conversations were digitally recorded and uploaded, the next step was transcribing the spoken words into written text. I want to thank two dedicated, excellent transcribers for their assistance in converting recordings into text files. Finally, I was able to transcribe the last few conversations myself using an app which I found at *www.transcribe.wreally.com*

In editing the transcriptions. I tried to be faithful to Sam's wording and meaning, and to capture exactly what he had in mind. To this end, I sought his opinion.

Here is a conversation we had about our collaboration.

Lenora: It's good to collect the stories as you recount them to me over the phone.

Sam: It is good. At this point, Lenora, it is really the only way I can do this.

Lenora: I know. Also I want your help as I work with the recordings and transcriptions.

Sam: Sure. What do you need?

Lenora: You know, Sam, the spoken word often requires editing before publication. I am trying to do this while keeping your words, but smoothing the language where necessary. At some point, I can read you a sample of what I've done, and you can judge for yourself.

Sam: I am very interested. Can you read me something right now, Lenora?

Lenora: I think so. Hang on a second while I get an edited story on the computer screen.

Sam: I am sitting here very patiently.

Lenora: Yes. Here is one of your stories. Tell me if I captured it correctly.

At this point, I read to Sam my edited version of "Another Frail Patient Story," a story in chapter 2, Tangling with the Orthopedists.

Lenora: That's it, Sam. What do you think?

Sam: Good job! You captured it all.

Lenora: Thanks. I tried to maintain the correct medical framework.

Sam: Yes, you did, Lenora. You did. I am really pleased.

Lenora: So glad to hear it, Sam.

Until the week before he died in February 2014, Sam continued to tell me his stories. I feel honored to bring them together in *Dr. Sam Sverdlik's Uncommon Stories.* I am only saddened that Sam did not live to see this work to fruition. It made both of us happy to be creating it together.

Wherever he is now, may he be smiling on the result!

Lenora Ucko   2015

2. Beginnings

I wanted to be a dentist.

Sam: I had always planned to go to dental school. I loved working with my hands - sculpting and carving - even as a 12-year-old. And so I felt dentistry was a nice field for me. That was what I kept touting.

Lenora: What changed your mind?

Sam: My father. He had other ideas. He would say to me every now and then, "For the same four years, you can get a medical degree. And wherever you go in the world, wherever you go as a doctor, you will be able to make a living."

Remember, Lenora, this was during the Hitler era, and in many places things were not open to Jews. Even in this country, there were unspoken quotas for Jews in medical schools. Anyway I was persuaded and applied to medical schools. I did. I applied to I don't know to how many. I was accepted by one!

Lenora: Only one?

Sam: Yes, that is all. And that was a medical school in Scotland. I was all set. I had my passport. I had contacted a rooming house in Scotland. I was in touch with others who were going to Scotland to medical school, and I was actually looking forward to going there.

Lenora: What stopped you?

Sam: My father intervened once again. He called me up one day and said, "I made an appointment up in Albany to see Dr. So and So, who is in charge of approving overseas medical education for New York State. I would like you to go with me and talk to him." I said, "Fine."

Lenora: What were you doing at the time?

Sam: I was working as a clerk at the Ice Company that summer, and I had to ask for time off. They all knew my Dad because he had worked for them in the past, and they said, "Sure, go ahead."

Lenora: And so you went?

Sam: Yes. In Albany, we met with this nice guy, someone important in the NYS Department of Education. At one point he turned to my father, saying, "Why would you let this man go to Scotland? There is going to be a war over there." My father asked, "Have you any suggestions?"

And the man promptly replied, "Yes. I went to a small college in upstate New York. I arrived there with five dollars in my pocket and a suitcase of clothing. And I left with five dollars and a suitcase of clothing, and a bachelor's degree. But I was able to get scholarships for a Ph.D. I suggest that your son go up there, do well for a year or two, and they will help get him into an American medical school."

Lenora: I bet you did not expect that.

Sam: No I didn't. It was a surprise. Then my father turned to me, "What do you think?" My answer was, "I'll buy it."

Lenora: And that worked out?

Sam: Yes. And that's how I got to Alfred University. I had been a degree candidate at William and Mary, in Virginia, but left there for Alfred. I never got to Scotland. But I still have the passport.

Lenora: An interesting story.

Sam: My Dad was unbelievable the way he influenced my choices. It was life-saving for me.

Hahnemann Medical College

Sam: As a medical student at Hahnemann Medical College, now part of Drexel University in Philadelphia, I was always in the top third of the class.

Lenora: Not a bad place to be.

Sam: I remember that during my first or second year there, my roommate asked me to tell him about Dr. Seidlin. I said, "What the hell do you know about Dr. Seidlin?" It turned out my roommate worked in the dean's office at Hahnemann to make an extra nickel for medical school expenses, and he was going through the charts of everyone in our class. In my chart, he found the strangest letter of recommendation. It was from Dr. Seidlin, who was a professor of mathematics at Alfred University. I had covered my ass by majoring in math, so that if necessary, I might become a math teacher. Dr. Seidlin wrote about me, "I highly recommend Sam Sverdlik. I know he will be a good math teacher. But Sam is certain that he will be a better doctor."

Lenora : Great recommendation!

Sam: I never got a chance to thank Seidlin. Dr. Seidlin has since passed away. But some years ago, I went to a reunion at Alfred University, and there was Seidlin's son. I went up and shared this story with him. His response was, "That sounds just like my father."

MIT training

Lenora : Speaking of math, I know at one point you received some special training at the Massachusetts Institute of Technology (MIT).

Sam: That was after graduating from medical school and after the war (World War II). I had decided to set up an office in general medical practice. I was referred to a well-known medical supply store in New York City where I went to get an examining table and other things I needed. "What about electronic equipment?" the salesman asked. "For what?" I wondered. His answer, "For diathermy treatment, of course." Surprised, I remarked, "I don't know the first damn thing about it." He answered, "We will show you." "No." I said, "No salesman is going to show me how to treat a patient."

Lenora: And that was the end of that, Sam?

Sam: No, it wasn't. I became very curious and wanted to find out more about diathermy equipment.

Lenora: And you did?

Sam: It turned out that soon thereafter, I attended meetings of the American Medical Association in New York. There I located the section on physical medicine. I walked over to the Information Desk and asked, "Where can I get training in how diathermy works and how to use electronic equipment?" This guy looked at me skeptically and asked, "What makes you think you can handle it?" I said, "I don't know." "Well," he was still skeptical. "How much math have you had?" I told him, "Differential equations and integral equations. I was going to be a math teacher." That did it. He took me by the arm and waltzed over me to another desk, saying, "Kurt, I want you to meet Dr. Sverdlik. He is acquainted with differential and integral equations in mathematics."

Lenora: And you talked to Kurt about math and diathermy treatment?

Sam: No. Not really. Kurt looked up at me and asked my name. I said, "Sverdlik." "Spell it," he said. And I did. To my surprise, he asked, "Do you have a relative who was visiting Europe before the war (World War II)?" I said, "It must be my uncle, Aaron." "And he had a friend in Germany at the time?" I tried to remember. "Would that be Max Brinks, a very successful German businessman who owned a castle in Wiesbaden." "Yes, that's the guy! That's the guy who helped me get to this country." Kurt and I suddenly became buddies.

Lenora: What a coincidence!

Sam: That wasn't all. Then Kurt added, "How would you like to go to MIT?" Amazed, I said, "Are you kidding?" "No, not at all," he assured me.

Lenora: That's how you learned about the MIT program?

Sam: Yes. And I was intrigued.

Lenora: I can understand that. Then what happened?

Sam: I asked Kurt what that was all about. He said, "This is a (Bernard) Baruch fellowship to train medical doctors in techniques and equipment in physical medicine. If you apply, I have every reason to believe you will be accepted."

Lenora: Could you change your other plans at that point?

Sam: Oh, yes. I was ready. I just said, "Okay, tell me what to do."

Lenora: Was there much preparation?

Sam: There was some. Among other things, I had to go back to my high school to get my records. This was September, and I stood on line with the high school kids who were waiting to have their programs changed. We were all impatient. But I finally got the records.

Lenora: What did your family think of all of this?

Sam: I don't remember. In any case, it wasn't an issue. And I was eager to be a part of that program. The next thing I knew I was going to MIT.

Lenora: What was that like?

Sam: Every Monday morning I left New York for Cambridge, Mass. and came home every Friday night. I was in a group with three other guys, one was the president of the American Academy of Physical Medicine, another a professor of physiology at the University of Kansas Medical School, and the third a practitioner. The undergraduates at MIT would stand in the hall, point at us and say, "Those are doctor doctors."

Lenora: What did you think of the MIT program?

Sam: It was great. The first day of class, I showed up with a slide rule (these were the days before the computer). This surprised everyone. Why did I have one, they wanted to know. I said, "We are learning all kinds of stuff in electronics and mathematics. Of course you need a slide rule." Now I was some kind of genius and my stock went up.

Introduction to Rehabilitation

Sam: While I was at MIT, there was a typhoid scare in New York. I called my wife to get a lot of the anti-toxin for injections. During my next weekend in New York, I made something like $30 or $40 (a lot of money in those days for one weekend's work) giving injections to prevent typhoid. When I came back to MIT, I was boasting about my accomplishment.

Lenora: And did that impress your colleagues?

Sam: I'm not sure. That's when the president of the American Academy of Physical Medicine called me aside and said, "Sam, never let money influence what you are going to do in medicine."

"What are you getting at?" I asked. He answered, "Don't go back into general practice. Continue with your training."

"For what?" I said. He told me, "We need guys like you in physical medicine."

Lenora: Did he mean rehabilitation, Sam?

Sam: Yes. But at that time, they were not yet using the word "rehabilitation."

Lenora: So what did he suggest?

Sam: That's what I said, "So what do you suggest?" He said, "Go to see Howard Rusk at Bellevue Hospital in New York City and work with him."

Lenora: Did you know much about Howard Rusk and his program?

Sam: No, not much. But that is what I did.

Lenora: And the rest is history.

Sam: Yes. The rest is history.

Lenora: Did you ever go back to general practice?

Sam: No, I did not. When I got back to New York after the MIT training, I went to work at Bellevue Hospital with Dr. Howard Rusk, the director of a brand new program in physical medicine and the first in the city. It was a natural transition since Rusk's program was also underwritten by the philanthropist, Bernard Baruch, the one who had provided the fellowship to MIT.

Meeting Barnard Baruch

Lenora: Did you ever meet Bernard Baruch?

Sam: Yes. He was quite a character.

Lenora: Tell me about it.

Sam: One day, Bernard Baruch came to visit us at Bellevue Hospital. The director, Howard Rusk, told me, "Stay with him." So I stayed with him. We were walking around, and all of a sudden he said, "Young man!" He had this high-pitched voice. I said, "Yes, Mr. Baruch?" But then he spotted Howard Rusk, who promptly ran over to him. Rusk also said. "Yes, Mr. Baruch?"

Pointing to a young patient from South America, Baruch asked, "How come this young man is here? I thought this hospital was only for the sick and poor of the City of New York." And this kid was from Venezuela, or someplace. Rusk could not answer that question, so he turned to me, "Yes, Sam. How come?" For a moment, I was startled. Then I remembered. "He is being covered by the Polio Foundation. They sent him up here. That's how we handle such cases."

Lenora: So, Sam, you saved Rusk's hide?

Sam: Yes. But there is one thing that I still feel bad about.

Lenora: What was that?

Sam: I had gotten this Baruch fellowship to go to MIT. And then when Bernard Baruch was visiting us, I did not say, "Thank you" to him. In retrospect, I say to myself, "Schmuck, why did you not thank Baruch for the fellowship that sent you to MIT? I low could you have missed that opportunity?"

Lenora: Well, Sam, you can't win them all. Sometimes things get away.

Sam: Yes, I know. But here it is 50, 60 years later, and I still go over it. To this day it niggles me.

Lenora: I can understand that. It would have been nice.

Sam: Yes, it would.

Working with Dr. Howard Rusk at Bellevue Hospital

Lenora: You were one of Howard Rusk's first trainees?

Sam: Yes. I was in at the beginning. There were also other guys there from all over the country.

Lenora: And Rusk was training the whole group?

Sam: Yes. But I was the only one that had some background in physics. So I was considered the scientific marvel. Especially in electronics, about which none of the others understood a damn thing.

Lenora: That MIT program must have been very helpful.

Sam: Yes. It was a one semester special program for physicians run by the Austrian physicist at MIT, Kurt Lyons. It turned out he was my "buddy" from the AMA meetings in New York.

Lenora: It's a small world.

Sam: You can say that again. Many years later, my wife and I came across his name in a curious way. At one point we were traveling in Europe. In Rome, we heard there was a Jewish Museum. So we went.

Lenora: Oh, I never heard of that museum.

Sam: It was a cockamamie museum. They didn't have much of anything. But they did have framed letters on the wall. And there was a letter from Kurt Lyons to the Jewish community in Rome, thanking them for the aid they gave him in getting to America during the Holocaust years.

Lenora: What a coincidence!

Sam: I will never forget it. When I saw his name, I let out a yell. "My God! It is a small world!"

At St. Vincent's Hospital

Lenora: I don't think we talked about how you got the job at St. Vincent's Hospital. What happened there, Sam?

Sam: Oh, St. Vincent's. In my last year as chief resident in the Rehabilitation Department at Bellevue/ NYU Hospital, I was sitting in the office of the Director of the Department, Howard Rusk, when his telephone rang. He answered it, and I heard him say, "I'll get back to you."

When he hung up, he turned to me. "Sammy," he said. He usually called me Sammy or SammyBoy. "They are setting up a Department of Rehab Medicine at St. Vincent's Hospital and are looking for a Director. SammyBoy, I think it's a good spot for you." My immediate reaction was, "If you say so, Chief, I'll take it." He called right back and told them, "I've got the man for you." And that's how I got the job.

Lenora: What a difficult job hunt!

Sam: Well, I did have to go down and be interviewed by the Director of Surgery.

Lenora: And I assume that went well?

Sam: Yes, very well. He was a nice guy, and he shepherded me through the early stages at St. Vincent's. Then the nuns got behind me and they backed me up 100%. A few minor diversions occurred when one or two doctors tried to make a stink over pretty much nothing. I remember one of the nuns cautioning one of them, "Back off, Jack!" The nuns kept these guys in line.

Lenora: Did you ever look for another job?

Sam: No, I didn't have to. It was a very, very rewarding job at St. Vincent's for forty years. I really did good work there - if I say so myself!

Lenora: Along the lines of doing a good job, I remember that years ago when I visited you at St. Vincent's, I noticed that you had shelves and shelves full of gifts that patients had given you.

Sam: Oh, I really had a unique position at St. Vincent's, I built a department that started out very small with very few resources and little space; and I ended up with a first class department in terms of resources and staff. I was getting visitors from all over the country who came to see my department and to verify firsthand the stories that were coming out about me.

Lenora: What about the gifts on the shelves behind the desk in your office, Sam?

Sam: Don't ask me to recount what they were. Right now, I can't remember. But I do remember the food. One patient would send me Greek cookies, along with donuts. A shipment came in regularly. I would keep them in the office and share them with my staff. Occasionally I would find a cake on my desk. Then we would all have it at lunchtime. Patients couldn't do enough to make me happy, and nothing gave me more pleasure. I felt I was giving the patients the best that I had, and they were giving me something in return. I enjoyed it all.

Lenora: Sounds great, and well deserved. These are good stories, Sam. Have you thought of others?

Sam: I do think of them, Lenora, and there are a lot of them. I keep saying to myself, "Get that pad and jot them down." But I don't do it.

Lenora: I know.

Sam: Incidentally, I remember asking you, do you have some good stories of your own and are you writing them down?

Lenora: No, I'm not.

3. Tangling With the Orthopedists

Sam: Dealing with orthopedists could be a bit tricky.

Lenora: How so?

Sam: There is a pecking order in medicine where the orthopedists rank higher than rehab specialists. Incidentally, many other specialties also rank closer to the top.

Lenora: Why isn't rehab higher on the list?

Sam: I don't know. I think maybe there isn't enough blood in it.

Lenora: Did that bother you?

Sam: No, it didn't. We worked with patients when these other guys were finished with them. At that point, we were critical in their recovery.

A Difference of Opinion

Lenora: Getting back to the orthopedists, what was your experience with them?

Sam: Here's an example. Usually, when I made rounds at the hospital, I had staff members who followed me around. One day, we stopped by a patient that the orthopedist had sent to us a while back for rehabilitation follow up. It was an interesting case.

Lenora: Please tell me about it.

Sam: This was an elderly woman who had fractured the small bone in her leg. It was healing nicely and she was walking. We were about ready to discharge her, when she fell and sustained another fracture.

Lenora: Oh, no!

Sam: Yes. I immediately put through a consultation call to the orthopedist. When I explained what happened, he said "Put her back in bed."

Lenora: And that's what you did?

Sam: Actually if I did that, she would be lying in bed for another six or eight weeks to wait for that thing to heal again. That did not seem necessary.

Lenora: How come?

Sam: It was a minor bone fracture and she could put weight on that leg without pain.

Lenora: What did you prescribe?

Sam: Then I told my staff that putting her back into bed seemed to me the dumbest thing we could do. My staff looked at me in disbelief. "What do we do now?" they asked. My answer was, "We don't do it. We just continue to work with this patient. She doesn't need bed rest." I prescribed having her walk to the extent that she could and resting afterward.

Lenora: And she got better and continued to walk?

Sam: The leg healed, and we didn't have to keep her in bed or tie up a bed for several weeks. The patient went home, and was able to walk on her own. It was really something.

Lenora: She must have been a very happy patient.

Sam: Oh, she was. But it was unheard of for a guy in rehab not to do what an orthopedist recommended. That word got around and for the next several weeks, almost every week a resident from another hospital came down to make rounds with me. They wanted to see the rehab guy who had stood up to the orthopedist and didn't back down. And of course I was right.

Lenora: And the orthopedist?

Sam: The orthopedist apparently felt he had to prescribe bed rest for an ankle fracture. But I didn't have to follow his prescription. And the orthopedist never lifted a finger.

Lenora: What did others think?

Sam: This incident gave me credibility for a long time. Residents from Cornell, Columbia, all the other programs in the city started to show up to take a look at this guy Sverdlik who contradicted the orthopedist. They wanted to see what I was running at St. Vincent's.

Lenora: Quite a reputation!

Sam: At that point, it was astonishing. It worked to my advantage, of course. I enjoyed the boost in esteem that I and my department had earned. I liked that.

Lenora: Well deserved, too.

Sam: It was a professional coup, Lenora.

Obstructions

Lenora: Was that your main brush with orthopedists?

Sam: Not really. You see, we had rehab programs at various hospitals, and particularly at teaching hospitals where there were orthopedic programs. From time to time, orthopedists there tended to be condescending to us and tried to put us in a bad light. Even at St Vincent's, they could be uncooperative.

Lenora: Like what?

Sam: Well, one of the tricks they sometimes tried was to wait until Friday afternoon to ask us suddenly to provide a physical therapist every day over the weekend. That could put my department in a bind. But I had alerted my staff that we may be faced with that kind of request and to be ready for it.

Lenora: Sounds like good planning.

Sam: Well, it's still not easy to find people at the last minute. This is often an unspoken rivalry between the orthopedists and rehabilitation.

Lenora: What do you mean?

Sam: For example, one Friday afternoon just before a holiday weekend,

I got a message from my administrator, Sister Carole (not her real name), who warned me, "You are going to get a call any minute to go down to see Sister (meaning the Head Nun)."

Lenora: Did that bother you?

Sam: First I had to know what was going on. "So, what's up?" I asked my administrator. Sister Carole told me that the orthopedist insisted on a therapist for his patient every day over the holiday weekend. "What's the status of that?" I persisted, "How do we handle it?" Nonchalantly, Sister Carole replied, "We worked it out already. We scheduled a therapist to come in on Saturday, Sunday, and Monday. Don't worry about it." Great. Now I could go down to see the Head Nun.

Lenora: How did that go?

Sam: Fine. She may have suspected that the orthopedist was trying to torpedo me. He had visited the Head Nun to insist that it was absolutely imperative that this patient, who he had kept in bed for about two or three weeks, receive intensive therapy every day. He wanted the Head Nun to see that it got done.

Lenora: Then what?

Sam: Sure enough, when I walked into the office, Sister said, "Will you be able to treat this patient every day this weekend?" "It's all taken care of, Sister," I assured her. That was the end of that. Except that the orthopedist lost some credibility. We had finessed his game.

Lenora: What was his reaction?

Sam: Well, for several years, he kept giving me a hard time.

Lenora: What did you do about that?

Sam: Nothing.

Lenora: Nothing?

Sam: That's right. After a while, he got over it. Then he and I became chummy and shared drinks and that sort of thing.

Lenora: What was his title?

Sam: He was the Director of Orthopedics.

Another Frail Patient Story

Lenora: Don't you have another "frail patient" story?

Sam: Oh yes. It had to do with this delightful, but very stubborn patient, an elderly woman, who was recovering from a fracture of the hip. At her age, the accident had been quite a shock.

The orthopedist had set the fracture and that finished his part of her care. He then sent her to us to return her to health.

Lenora: Sounds like a challenge.

Sam: Yes, it was. It was slow and difficult. However, after several weeks, she was at the stage of restoring movement, standing, taking weight on the affected leg and ready to walk. After a thorough physical examination that showed the hip was sufficiently recovered, I prescribed a series of physical therapy sessions.

Lenora: And that speeded her recovery?

Sam: Not so fast. Not so fast. Little did I realize how difficult that was going to be! After several days and many attempts by the physical therapists in my department, I was told that there was no way this woman could be enticed to take the first step. They had tried everything in the book. Sadly, nothing worked.

Lenora: Then what?

Sam: Apparently it was time for the Big Doctor (me) to try his luck (skill?). I went up to the gymnasium where we had the parallel bars. The elderly woman was standing between the bars, clutching them tightly with both hands. Right next to her, a physical therapist was urging, cajoling, gently helping. But the woman would have none of it. She did not budge. The physical therapist turned to me in despair and whispered, "I can't get her to do a damn thing."

Lenora: So what did you do?

Sam: So in all my dignity, I walked up to the parallel bars and introduced myself to the woman. Then I said pleasantly, "Can I see you take a few steps?"

Lenora: And did she try?

Sam: No, of course not. Instead, she gave me a withering look, and in a patronizing tone announced. "Doctor, I am 84 years old!"

Lenora: What could you say to that?

Sam: Without thinking, I smiled and burst out, "So what the hell do you want, a medal?"

Lenora: How very professional of you!

Sam: Perhaps not. But she started to laugh out loud and then she took off!

Lenora: You mean she took her first steps?

Sam: Yes! She just needed a little shaking up and my response did it. You know if I had thought about my answer in advance, I might not have said that. But it was spontaneous - and it worked!

Lenora: What a saga!

Sam: I love that story!

Lenora: So do I.

4. Pseudo-Psychiatry at St. Vincent's

Lenora: You told me that at St. Vincent's Hospital, at one time you took on the role of a psychiatrist with some patients. Would you tell me more about that?

Sam: Oh, that role? Lord, yes.

Lenora: Do you remember working with a nun as a patient?

The Nun's Story

Sam: Oh yeah. This is the way that came about. Sister Anne (not her real name), who taught at a local parochial school, was plagued with backaches. She was first sent to the neurologist; then to the orthopedist; then to the rheumatologist; and then they finally sent her to me for rehabilitation. I recognized immediately that she needed psychiatric intervention. I tried to get her to buy it, but she wasn't buying.

Lenora: Was this all for her backaches?

Sam: Well, no. She actually called herself "the masturbating nun." She kept saying, "How do I get rid of this obsession?" I told her "I have no idea how you get rid of it, but a good psychiatrist would help." "No! No! No!" she cried.

Lenora: Quite a challenge! How did you handle it?

Sam: I consulted the psychiatrist at the hospital.

Lenora: Did that help?

Sam: I'm not sure. He suggested I keep meeting with Sister Anne and continue to talk with her. I told him I didn't think I was up to that.

Lenora: And that took care of the situation?

Sam: Not at all. Then the psychiatrist said, "All you have to do is come to us after each session and we'll tell you how to go from there."

Lenora: What did you think?

Sam: I was skeptical. But the psychiatrist kept saying it would work.

Lenora: Did it?

Sam: I guess for a while. After each appointment with Sister Anne, I would see the psychiatrist the very next morning. I would then spill out everything that the Sister was telling me, and what my responses were. The psychiatrist would say, "You're doing fine, Sam. Keep it up. Keep it up."

Lenora: What were the sessions like?

Sam: The nun often came in to our appointments with letters that were 10 to 12 pages long. She was a high school teacher, very, very articulate and comfortable expressing herself. And she would write in the horniest way you ever could imagine. These letters were really amazing.

Lenora: What would you do with them?

Sam: I would read them over carefully, reinsert them in the envelope, and the next time I saw her, I would hand them back to her. She was a hot shot when it came to her imaginary sex life. And she had me as one of her partners a fair amount of the time. I would read that but I wouldn't respond to it. I would however share it with the psychiatrist with whom I shared everything from our sessions. He kept saying, "You're doing fine, Sam. Just keep it up, keep it up."

Lenora: Were you finally comfortable with the arrangement?

Sam: I don't think so. Every time I told the psychiatrist, "This isn't enough for her. You have to get me out of this. I'm not up to it," he always answered, "No, no! We can't do that. You can't leave her; that's abandoning her. You've got to stay with it." So I stayed.

Lenora: And all this time you were getting help from the psychiatrist?

Sam: Yes. But then one morning I came in early to tell him about an episode from the afternoon before. The guy said to me, "This is the last one, Sam." "What do you mean this is the last one?" I asked. He smiled and answered, "If you can't do this now on your own, you'd better take up another profession." And from then on, I had to do it without the backup of a psychiatrist.

Lenora: How did that go?

Sam: It went OK. And that's how I became a pseudo-psychiatrist!

Lenora: What happened with Sister Anne?

Sam: After a while I somehow got Sister Anne to accept the idea of consulting a certified psychiatrist. I never found out whether she got rid of her problem. But the way I solved my role in this was to send her to another doctor.

Lenora: Quite a story!

Sam: I guess so.

Dealing with Pain

Lenora: Were there other patients with whom you did "pseudo-psychiatric" work or that the psychiatrist sent to you?

Sam: No, no, the psychiatrist didn't send me patients. Patients came to me through more normal channels. They would present a physical problem, first to the internist who checked them out and sent them to the orthopedist. The orthopedist checked them out and sent them to the rheumatologist. Then the rheumatologist checked them out and sent them to me. When they got to me that was the end of the line. I had no place to send them unless I thought they needed a psychiatrist.

Lenora: Were there other patients with whom you acted as the pseudo-psychiatrist or was it just Sister Anne?

Sam: Oh, I would say that easily the majority of low back pain cases, maybe 60 %, are psychosomatic. And nobody attempted to talk the patients out of it, except me.

Lenora: What was the psychiatrists' role in these cases?

Sam: The psychiatrists wanted no part of it. They would tell me, "You know how to handle it, Sam. Why don't you take care of this patient."

And so I accepted the challenge. I worked with a fair number of patients with low back pain and had a bit of success. Not in every case, of course. But I did get many people with chronic complaints to be pain free and to return to work.

Lenora: How do you explain your success where patients with chronic pain became pain-free.

Sam: Pain is a psychological activity of your mind. You perceive pain in your brain. That's where you judge it as severe or tolerable or intolerable. With those as givens, it is my contention that in many cases, pain can come under the patient's control. And the degree to which pain compromises behavior is also under one's control.

Lenora: How come?

Sam: For example. there are cases where medically the patient has fully recovered, but the perception of pain lingers in the brain. Here the doctor can help the patient recognize and remove the perception and return to a normal life.

Lenora: That sounds like a different view of pain.

Sam: Well, I have been using this approach for many, many years with a good degree of benefit and with a great many people. After a while, these patients began to see that they were in control and nobody else was. With some, the pain went away entirely and they went back to work.

Lenora: Sounds great.

Sam: Well, remember this does not apply to everyone. Medical conditions can give rise to accompanying pain. And the doctor needs to recognize the difference.

Lenora: Do other doctors use your approach?

Sam: I'm not sure. Some probably do, but many do not. Often patients get doctors to write prescriptions and make recommendations, which many times are of no benefit at all.

5. Teaching and Training

Lenora: You told me that you had done a lot of teaching and training.

Sam: Oh, my God, yes. Yes, I trained I don't know how many people and on at various levels. I had a very active teaching and training program. And 99% was all on my back. I never realized that I was carrying so much.

Lenora; How did all that come about?

Sam: It seemed to mushroom as the need arose. I was asked to train therapists at Bellevue Hospital and at other hospitals. I also taught students at New York University. I set up rehab departments at other hospitals. I would create programs and implement them. These were responsibilities I assigned to myself. I busted my ass, but I didn't realize it.

Lenora: And you trained staff for other hospitals that were starting rehab departments?

Sam: Oh. Very much so.

Lenora: Can you name some of the hospitals where you set up programs?

Sam: Of course. St. Vincent's in New York. Then there was St. Vincent's in Staten Island and St Vincent's in Yonkers. St Joseph's Hospital in Far Rockaway, Rockaway Beach Hospital, and Long Beach Memorial Hospital. And then there was Danbury General Hospital that I can tell you about at a later time. There may have been more, but I can't think of them right now. But that's not a bad record.

Lenora: Not bad at all.

Sam: Each time I was asked to start a department at another hospital, I wanted to help and I would. For an initial period, I was the department with a therapist and a nurse. We would come once a week and the patients would be lined up waiting for us. Things usually ran well. But after a while, it reached the point where I couldn't

31

handle so much. I was overwhelmed by the amount of work I was piling on myself, and I had to give some of it up.

Lenora: Tell me about your teaching at New York University.

Sam: Well, I taught at different levels. At the undergraduate level, I would go down to New York University at Washington Square, usually twice a week and lecture college students on physical therapy. After a while, I arranged for the students to come to me. We met in classrooms at the School of Nursing.

Lenora: And at the NYU medical school?

Sam: Well I'd say that at the medical school things were thriving, and I was in the middle of it all with a lot of responsibilities.

Lenora: Can you explain that?

Sam: The medical students would come to me at St. Vincent's Hospital, twice a week for a full year - two semesters

Lenora: How did that work?

Sam: At 4 o'clock, we would clear the department for the medical students. From 4 to 6, I taught them various aspects of rehabilitation medicine, including the use of equipment. Then for the next two hours, they would practice on each another.

Lenora: Quite a load you were carrying.

Sam: Remember, I also had a training program for new residents in my own department. That too required lectures and demonstrations at the hospital, and training in the use of equipment.

Lenora: And in your spare time?

Sam: Funny you should ask. Over the years, I wrote several professional papers. For some, I was the sole author and others were coauthored. The articles were published in journals like the Journal of the American Medical Association, the Journal of the Rehabilitation Society, and the New York State Journal of Medicine.

Lenora: Impressive!

Sam: I must say I had a very effective program. People came from all over to listen to my lectures. I had a good reputation. And I never realized how good I was. I just handled whatever came along, and did it mostly alone.

Lenora: I imagine you could have moved up to larger medical establishments and higher income brackets.

Sam: I was aware of that. However, I ran a good department. I was a very competent therapy guy, and I was a good teacher. And I recognized that that was enough. I didn't need any more. Getting into higher levels didn't particularly attract me. And I survived.

Lenora: I think you did more than survive.

Sam: I would say so.

Lenora: I would say you were a startling success.

Sam: Well, I wouldn't go that far. But I know that I was highly respected. People who trained with me were able to get good positions all over the country.

Lenora: That must have pleased them.

Sam: Oh yes. Whenever they would run into me, they'd always turn to the other person in the group and say "This is Sam, the person who taught me everything I know about rehabilitation." It was quite a compliment.

Lenora: My guess is that you taught them not only about rehabilitation, but about relating to patients on a personal level.

Sam: You see, I didn't have a lab. I didn't have a physiologist or a psychologist or other support staff that other departments had. I had to rely on my own clinical skills. And I developed protocols on how to examine a patient, how to motivate a patient, how to evaluate if therapy was working or not.

Lenora: A foresighted approach, Sam. Today these issues are receiving more and more attention.

Sam: For me, they were the bread and butter elements of a good program. The people who trained with me recognized that. When they talked to guys from other programs, these others were amazed at how realistic were the guys who trained with me.

6. Hidden Valley Project for Handicapped Children

How it started

Lenora: Can you tell me about the Hidden Valley Project. As I remember, it is an unusual story.

Sam: Okay, I can do that. The Hidden Valley Project originated through an unforeseen sequence of events.

Lenora: Unforeseen?

Sam: Well, yes. To begin with, not only was I the Director of Rehabilitation at St. Vincent's Hospital in New York City, but also at St. Vincent's Hospital in Yonkers.

Lenora: And the one in Yonkers had to do with Hidden Valley?

Sam: No. Not really. It's just that the one in Yonkers was situated next door to the Catholic Charities Recreation Building where there was a swimming pool. And that made all the difference.

Lenora: In what way?

Sam: One Spring day many years ago, I was examining some handicapped children at the Yonkers facility. It occurred to me that if Catholic Charities allowed the kids to use the pool, I could then prescribe it as part of their therapy.

Lenora: Not a bad idea.

Sam: No, not at all. And so I went over and spoke to them about this.

Lenora: Was it a problem for them?

Sam: On the contrary, they were very cooperative and willing to help.

Lenora: How did it work out?

Sam: It was great. The kids were happy to be in the pool, and I kept track of how they were doing. This went on through the Spring, and the kids were benefiting.

A Look to the Future

Sam: One day the mother of one of the children came to me and said: "What are you doing for the kids for the summer?" Surprised, I blurted out, "Are you kidding? What do you mean what am I doing for the kids for the summer?"

She insisted, "Don't they deserve to go to camp in the summer?"

"Of course they do," I replied. "But why are you making it my problem?"

She simply said: "Because I want you to take care of it."

I had to tell her that was not possible. "I can't," I said, "but maybe you can do it."

Lenora: What made you say that?

Sam: I don't know. But it turned out that she was the wife of a reporter for The New York Herald Tribune, and when she returned with her child the next week, she had good news.

Lenora: What was it?

Sam: "I talked to my husband," she told me, "and he talked to some of the people at the Herald Tribune." Apparently, the newspaper, as part of its Fresh Air Fund program, was running summer camping for poor kids. The mother continued, "They have a camp site we could use. Toward the end of the summer when the regular camping program is over, we can have the facilities for one week for our children."

Lenora: Could you run a whole camping program, Sam?

Sam: No. But somehow that mother and the Fresh Air Fund had figured it out. The people in the camp kitchen volunteered to stay there for another week to do the cooking. And the parents of the kids were prepared to act as counselors and to take care of whatever else was involved.

Starting an Annual Program

Sam: And that is how we adapted Hidden Valley as a camp for handicapped children.

Lenora: How long did it last?

Sam: Would you believe from that time to this day. It became a permanent project sponsored by the Fresh Air Fund. The Fund designated a couple of their camps to accept handicapped kids. We made sure that those camps did not have steep hills or staircases to climb or other obstacles. Then we were able to accommodate I don't know how many children every summer.

Lenora: That's impressive.

Sam: Oh, I insisted on another thing with the Fresh Air Fund people. The encampments were usually for two weeks at a time. I said: "That is not enough." They said: "That's how we have been doing it for years - two weeks." I said: "But not with handicapped children. You have got to give them a little extra time." And so we were able to extend the camp time for them for three weeks!

Lenora: Anything else?

Sam: Yes. At a few other Fresh Air Fund camps, we were able to integrate handicapped children into the regular camp group. It worked fine. We had no trouble.

Lenora: And now?

Sam; I believe the Fresh Air Fund still has these camps going on. For years, I was involved in visiting the camps, examining the kids, and making sure things were going OK.

Lenora: What a wonderful thing you did for so many handicapped children!

Sam: If you want to put it that way, I won't argue with you. Lenora, would you like to hear an unusual experience I had one day, when visiting one of the camp sites?

Lenora: Of course I would.

A remarkable recovery

Sam: I was standing at the side of the pool where the children were frolicking. I was watching this little girl whom I knew. She had had polio and it affected her legs. Now I saw her kicking her legs under water.

Lenora: Hardly what you expected.

Sam: That's right. I pulled her out of the pool and put her down at the side of the pool. I said, "Move your legs." She said, "I can't." I said, "Yes, you can." And she started to cry. I said, "Stop that and move your legs." Nothing happened.

Lenora: Then what?

Sam: I wiggled her toes. She thought that was funny. So I said, "Wiggle this toe" pointing to one. And goddamit, she wiggled that toe!

Lenora: What a breakthrough!

Sam: Yes. And I immediately said to her, "See, it's working. You can move your legs!"

Lenora: Did you have an audience around you by then?

Sam: No. Only her parents who came running over when they saw their child lying on the side of the pool.

Lenora: Why were the parents there?

Sam: They had come to the camp that day because they knew I was going to be there, and they wanted to talk with me. Now they were frightened. "What is the matter?" they gasped. "Nothing is the matter," I told them.

Lenora: A dramatic story!

Sam: Then I told the child, "Stand up." "I can't," she complained. But I said, "Yes, you can."

Lenora: You were persistent!

Sam: Well, before I was finished, she stood up and walked away, normally.

Lenora: That's amazing!

Sam: Yes, it was. It was a delight.

Lenora: And the parents?

Sam: Oh, the parents' jaws dropped. They expected to have a permanently handicapped child with a paralyzed leg. And it turned out that the leg had recovered, but the kid had continued to assume that it was still paralyzed.

Lenora: How do you explain that, Sam?

The Mind-Body Connection

Sam: This is not unusual for people with mild strokes and other conditions. I picked that up along the way. I never found anything about it in the books, although I never did a detailed survey of the literature. But after treating many different patients, I realized that this was not an unusual thing. With some people after an episode of some sort, they think paralysis is the final outcome. Then their body recovers, but their mind doesn't. And you just have to rewire them, so to speak. I did that a fair number of times with patients.

Lenora: What Is this called?

Sam: I don't know how to characterize it. To me it was all part of a day's work. I didn't stop to make any appraisal of how important it was. All I know is that I would occasionally get a patient that I recognized had recovered from a paralytic episode. But only I knew that. To the patient, that limb was still paralyzed. And you had to get them to recognize that it wasn't.

Lenora: And you didn't write that up for publication?

Sam: Exactly. I never wrote up any papers on these things. Perhaps I should have. I just did my thing.

Lenora: For you it was all in a day's work. But for your patients, it was a gift of a lifetime.

Sam: Oh, yes. Oh yes. I was aware of that. If I hadn't done it, some of them would have continued to assume they were permanently paralyzed. And they really weren't. They had recovered.

Lenora: Do you know whether this is now part of the assessment that doctors make in treating paralysis today?

Sam: No, I don't know. You know, I would, so to speak, find these insights, act on them within my practice, and relate them over a beer at a conference. And the other doctors would look at me and say, "Sam, why the hell do all of these unusual things happen to you and not to us."

Lenora: Yes, why?

Sam: After a while I finally came up with the answer. I said, "Because I keep talking to the patient. And I keep watching them." Then if I see that there's no atrophy of the leg and that the circulation is normal and that the nail growth is normal, then it isn't a paralyzed leg any more. And I just get the patient to start using the leg, under water or wherever. Then before long, they are riding a bicycle.

Lenora: Clearly, you have done wonders in so many people's lives.

Sam: Well, if you want to say that, that's your privilege. I never stopped to figure out where it sat in the spectrum of things. I just took it in stride and kept going. And I don't know how many times I would crack one of these things apart. And all of a sudden, a paralyzed arm or leg would be working.

Lenora: I am so glad to have this story.

Sam: Okay. You do with it as you see fit.

Today Camp Hidden Valley, one of five summer camps run by the Fresh Air Fund , is reserved for disabled and able-bodied boys and girls, 8 to 12 years old. The Fresh Air Fund is financed largely through donations solicited by The New York Times. At this unique camp, disabled children live and play with able-bodied boys and girls and find out how much they have in common. Hidden Valley campers have a variety of disabilities including sickle-cell anemia, cerebral palsy, muscular dystrophy, hearing impairments, emotional problems and physical handicaps that require the children to use wheelchairs, braces or crutches. At Camp Hidden Valley, disabled children dream of climbing mountains, learning to swim, laughing with new friends -- and they realize those dreams.

All because many years ago, Dr. Sam Sverdlik went next door to the Yonkers, NY Catholic Charities Recreation Building that had a swimming pool!

7. Happenings at St. Vincent's

Cardinal Spellman's Visit

Sam: One day, I was informed by the Head Nun that Francis Joseph Spellman, Cardinal of New York, was coming to visit the hospital, and he would be accompanied by Alfred P. Sloan of the Sloan-Kettering Cancer Institute. Would I set up something of interest to show my department's accomplishments.

Lenora: A challenge?

Sam: Well, I consulted my staff, and we decided to introduce the Cardinal and Mr. Sloan to five patients who were recovering from cancer surgery. I knew the visitors were especially interested in cancer treatment.

Lenora: Had the five patients suffered from different types of cancer?

Sam: No. The ones I selected all had had their larynxes removed. All had suffered cancer of the throat. They no longer had a voice box, but could speak through a prosthetic device. I would normally see them individually for treatment, but to meet the visitors, I had all five in my office at once.

When the Cardinal and his guest arrived, I introduced them to my staff. Then I presented the patients, and encouraged the Cardinal and Mr. Sloan to converse with each one. The visitors were surprised at how well the patients could communicate.

Lenora: Perhaps not what they expected.

Sam: Maybe. But something else surprised them more.

Lenora: What was that?

Sam: You see, these five patients were all foreign born. Even with their voice box removed, they continued to "speak" with a foreign accent. An Italian accent. A Jewish accent. An Irish accent. And so on, through the prosthetic device.

Lenora: I never thought of that. What is the explanation?

Sam: They didn't have a voice box, but the accent was in their brain. As I explained to the visitors, the voice box is the piano. The rest of the voice is in your head. That's how you play the piano and also what gives distinctiveness to your speech.

Lenora: Quite fascinating! What was the Cardinal's reaction?

Sam: I can't recall much. He was pleased of course. But I think I impressed Sloan of Sloan-Kettering even more. Yes, they said it was a good presentation. I didn't hear any more about it after that.

Negotiating with the Administration

Lenora: There's another story I would like you to tell. The one where you dealt with the Head Nun for furnishings for your office.

Sam: Oh, yes. After several months at St. Vincent's, I asked for a sofa for my office. It would be good for some patients. And I could use it to relax when necessary.

Lenora: Was that customary? Did other doctors have sofas in their office?

Sam: Many did. Especially department heads.

Lenora: And was there a problem?

Sam: Well, lots of delays and nothing happened. I finally went down to see the Head Nun. After listening to her recounting the financial bind they were in and the difficulty of making the arrangements, I looked at her and said quietly, "Sister, it hurts me to say this. But this sounds like anti-semitism to me."

The Sister was taken aback. "Oh, no," she said. "We can't have that!"

Before I knew it, there was a sofa in my office. I thought, I must remember this.

Sometime later, I felt my office could use an additional book shelf. Again I went down to see the Head Nun. And again there were financial and other constraints. I opened my mouth and began "Sister…" But this wise administrator smiled, reached over and patted my wrist. "Dr. Sverdlik," she said. "It worked once, but it won't work a second time." And it didn't.

The Sheriff Comes to my Office

Sam: One day, people from the Sheriff's office came to see me.

Lenora: At the hospital?

Sam: Yes, at St. Vincent's.

Lenora: What did they want?

Sam: They came in connection with my brother's handling of my father's estate and his law practice.

Lenora: What was that about?

Sam: It was a horror! We had had a series of family tragedies. First my father took sick and was ill for a long time. My brother went to law school at night, got a law degree, and worked in the law office. Then Dad died. My brother took over the law practice and was executor of the estate. And it's hard to believe, but within a short time, he ran both into the ground.

Lenora: How come?

Sam: I don't know. To cover the debts, he ended up borrowing vast sums of money from family members. And we all countersigned huge loans that he was taking out.

Lenora: How did your brother handle all that?

Sam: He didn't. We had another family tragedy. He developed leukemia and within a few months he was dead.

Lenora: What a sad turn of events!

Sam: Yes. Several family members, I included, found ourselves owing hundreds of thousands of dollars, and had no way of paying it back. We had to go into bankruptcy. It was awful.

Lenora: That was the reason the Sheriff came to your office?

Sam: Pretty much. I really thought they were coming for me.

Lenora: What did they want?

Sam: My first reaction was to put my hands out and say "Do you want to put the irons on?"

Lenora: Were you serious?

Sam: I don't know, maybe. But they laughed and answered, "Take it easy, Doc. Take it easy." "What is it that you want from me?" I persisted. They replied, "We're here to find out what you have in this office that we can attach, so we can pay the creditors." I told them, "You can't attach anything. I don't own this office. It all belongs to the hospital." That was largely true. "That's all we want to know." they told me. And they walked out.

Lenora: That was it?

Sam: Yes, that was it. I never saw them again.

8. Opportunities Elsewhere

Washington possibilities

Lenora: Would you say something about when you were invited to apply for positions in and around Washington, D.C.

Sam: Well, several medical facilities sought me out and solicited me, whether I was interested in applying for their job or not. One, for instance, was working at a major teaching hospital connected with Georgetown University. To be in Washington, D.C. or in Baltimore was the pinnacle in the field of rehabilitation. You were right close to the important buttons, and whoever occupied these positions was highly respected in the field. I apparently was in the running. But I often felt I didn't have anything compared to some of the other guys they were considering.

Lenora: But they solicited you. And did you apply?

Sam: Yes, I submitted applications, but I didn't count on getting the positions.

Lenora: Wasn't there also a solicitation from the National Institutes of Health.

Sam: Yes. Yes. There the guy in rehab medicine was retiring and he kept after me. "Sam," he kept reminding me, "I want you to apply for this job." He really wanted me to succeed him.

Lenora: Were you tempted?

Sam: I guess so. It was quite a compliment.

Lenora: And you applied?

Sam: Yes, I did. It was a sort of an ego trip to see if I would be offered the job.

Lenora: Were you?

Sam: No. I wasn't.

Lenora: How'd you feel about that?

Sam: Mixed feelings to be honest with you. Some disappointment, of course. But still, I am not a very political person. And I felt I would be getting into deeper waters than I could handle. I was just as happy that I didn't get it.

Lenora: Was your family impressed with the solicitations?

Sam: Oh, they were very happy with the outcome. You see, my wife and my mother were both very active in discouraging me. They didn't like the idea of a move to the Washington area.

Lenora: Really. Who finally got the position? Do you remember?

Sam: No I don't, but a very competent guy. You know it takes a certain quality to know how to flatter people, to make sure to show up at all the right occasions, and so on. I never felt at ease in that kind of environment.

Lenora: It is a whole different thing. It's both medical and political.

Sam: Yes. And I was actually handicapped. I didn't know how to deal with the politics. It's a skill that I don't have. I ran a good department. I was a very competent therapy guy, and I was a good teacher. That's sufficient. It didn't particularly attract me to get into some high political level. And I survived.

Danbury, Connecticut

Lenora: Was there ever a position that you really wanted?

Sam: Well, yes. There was one in Danbury, Connecticut.

Lenora: Danbury? I don't know about Danbury.

Sam: Let me tell you about it. One of my best friends was at Danbury General Hospital, and I was asked to create a rehab program there. It turned out to be a great experience.

Lenora: In what way? .

Sam: I built a marvelous program. It was unbelievable. Everyone I worked with was so cooperative, I didn't have to do anything but see the patients and write on the chart. I would also dictate my notes at the end of my sessions there, and when I'd come in the next week, they would be typed up and waiting for me. Then I'd edit and sign them. As far as billing was concerned, they took care of that, too. And they would pay their bill promptly. It was a beautiful operation. I should really have gone up there. I would have had a very good time.

Lenora: But you didn't go.

Sam: No. I finally gave it up. I was overburdened with both Danbury and my department at St. Vincent's. Driving up to Danbury every week was not a picnic. And in the wintertime it could be troublesome. It just became too much.

Lenora: Was there any alternative?

Sam: Well, I had a dream of moving to Danbury. I was set to move and live there and work there because I was having so much fun. But I never did.

Lenora: Why not?

Sam: My wife, mainly. She could not see living in Danbury, Connecticut, and was very much opposed to going there.

Lenora: And that was the end of Danbury?

Sam: Yes. I hated to give it up. It was a beautiful program.

Lenora: Disappointing.

Sam: Yes. And sad.

9. Three Aspects of Rehabilitation

A Bar Mitzvah Story

Lenora: I seem to remember a story you told me about a death at a celebration.

Sam: Oh, yes, yes. It was a Bar Mitzvah dinner, joyous and festive. I was invited and so were some of my medical colleagues. We sat together at the same table near an older couple whom we did not know. At one point, the husband excused himself to go to the men's room. And he dropped dead.

Lenora: What a shock!

Sam: Of course. Immediately all of us doctors rushed to the patient and tried to resuscitate him. Too late. The patient was gone.

Lenora: And then?

Sam: Well, nothing more to be done. Someone called for an ambulance. And all the doctors returned to the table. All, that is, except me.

Lenora: Why not you?

Sam: It took a while, but I finally rejoined the others. And they said to me, "What the hell were you doing all this time?" I said I was working with what was left.

Lenora: And they wanted to know what was left?

Sam: Yes. I said, "The widow." I sat with her a while, commiserated with her, and helped her compose herself. Then someone came and took her home.

Lenora: And the other doctors didn't think of that?

Sam: Apparently not. They only tried resuscitation, the theatrical stuff - which didn't work. And then they were finished. This gave me a chance to say, "In rehabilitation, we work with what's left after you guys are done with your dramatic interventions." I could have added that a good rehab program addresses each particular situation from many angles - not just the patient's physical condition, but also psychological, cultural, and family aspects. And they are different for each patient.

Lenora: Sounds like a broad vision of medical care.

Sam: Maybe that sums it up.

Malcolm Mahle's Story

Lenora: Sam, it seems to me there's another story you told me that illustrates what we're talking about. The rehabilitation of the young man who had many disabilities and could hardly get around. I think his name was Mal or something.

Sam: Oh, yes. Malcolm Mahle (not his real name). He was known as Mal.

Lenora: Can you tell me about him?

Sam: Sure. Mal was still a young man when he suffered a stroke at the base of his brain. It left him severely disabled. His fairly wealthy family looked for the best medical care they could find. Still whatever they found did not improve Mal's condition much. When someone suggested that they talk to me about rehabilitation, they first consulted their own doctor. Didn't he think that they ought to call in Dr. Sverdlik for a rehabilitation program? The learned doctor shook his head and said no, that would likely be a waste of time.

Lenora: But they called you anyway?

Sam: Yes. I don't know why. Maybe they thought rehab was worth a shot since nothing else was helping,

Lenora: What was that like for you?

Sam: Well, I finally got to see Mal. He was halfway between bedridden and chair ridden. He hardly walked at all. His speech was garbled, and his coordination was all out of whack.

Lenora: A lot of deficits! Was there much you could do?

Sam: I had to see further. Mal's father was usually present for the medical appointments. And I was able to enlist his father's help on occasion to try to improve Mal's walking. With his father holding him up on one side and I on the other, Mal could proceed a short way down the corridor and back. Then one day, a startling thing happened.

Lenora: What was that?

Sam: We were moving down the corridor a little further than usual and came to a step down. As we prepared to turn back, Mal stopped and said in his halting speech, "Wanna jump!" Mal's father froze. But I gave it a moment's thought, and then said, "OK, Mal, if you want to jump, we'll jump." And with Mr. Mahle on one side and I on the other, holding Mal tightly under the arms, the three of us jumped down the one step. Mr. Mahle was speechless. I was content. But Mal was delirious with joy!

Lenora: Was that a breakthrough?

Sam: You bet it was! After that, Mal felt he could do anything.

Lenora: And could he?

Sam: No, not anything. But enough to turn his life around.

Lenora: Please go on – what happened?

Sam: With lots, and I mean lots, of effort on his part and a great deal of encouragement and prescribed therapy on mine, Mal overcame his difficulties enough to lead a fairly normal life.

Lenora: He did?

Sam: Yes. He eventually was able to walk by himself with a cane. His garbled speech improved. His coordination remained a problem, but not so much that it interfered with what he wanted to do.

Lenora: And what did he want to do?

Sam: Oh, you know. He went back to school and completed his education. He found a job. He drove his own car. And best of all, he got married, had children, and had a good life.

Lenora: Wow - that's remarkable!

Sam: I was very proud of that.

Lenora: I don't blame you. You know, giving people back their life is an unbelievable gift.

Sam: Well, that was a big thing. Still I had to recognize that I didn't cure people of their disease. But they did get maximum benefit from treatment. They were still disabled, but they could function. I often would step in at a time when a great many patients, and their doctors, had given up, feeling the patients might never be able to do anything for themselves again. I would slowly nudge them along to where many would be living a pretty full life, driving a car, going back to business, and things like that.

Lenora: A wonderful contribution!

Sam: I had to tell myself that because that was not what the average doctor was doing.

Lenora: True. And you did it by working out individualized treatment? I'm trying to figure out what the mechanism was that got your patients to improve so much.

Sam: There was no mechanism because no two were alike really. Motivating the patient was the key. To get them to want to work at improvement, that took a lot of gentle encouragement. I would make a big fuss when they took a step or when they climbed a step or whatever.

Lenora: And it worked.

Sam: And it worked. Yes.

Lenora: That's the important thing - it worked.

Comparison with Others

Sam: Yes. But when I'd get together with medical colleagues who had graduated from medical school about the same time I did, there was a difference. These guys were earning big money, going on exotic vacations, making big investments. I never achieved that level of income, and for a long time, I even felt I was a failure, so to speak.

Lenora: Hard to believe.

Sam: And then I finally realized what I was doing for people. And rehabilitation medicine was never a big money making specialty, anyway.

Lenora: No it wasn't. But you were the one who achieved the greater success.

Sam: Yes. To that extent yes. After a while, I recognized that I was doing a unique job. I was running a great department. And best of all, patients were benefiting from my approach and my treatment. But it took a couple of years for me to get to that point.

Lenora: I guess it takes a while to sort it all out. Congratulations!

Sam: Thanks.

10. Epilogue

Retirement

Lenora: What was it like when you retired, Sam?

Sam: You know, Lenora, I had been at St. Vincent's for forty years. Almost all the people I had interacted with over the years, my staff people as well as colleagues in other departments – they were all gone, retired or moved elsewhere. It seems I was one of the last ones to go.

Lenora: And your department?

Sam: When I announced my retirement, the administration recruited new staff and a new director. I hardly knew them.

Lenora: Were you happy with that?

Sam: I don't know. But it was time for me to leave. I think the newcomers were just as happy to see me go, as I was to go. They would set the pace, and it would be different in the future.

Lenora: Did you have a Retirement Party?

Sam: Yes, but even that was rather sterile.

Lenora: Were you disappointed?

Sam: Yes, a little. But since 90% of the people who showed up had known me for only a short period of time, we hardly had much in common. There was no affection or even knowledge about me and my work, as there had been in the past. It's like we were all strangers.

Lenora: Were the Sisters, the nuns, there?

Sam: Yes, the nuns popped in. They were warmer and more personal. Some of them had known me a long time.

Lenora: And your going-away gift?

Sam: I think they gave me something, but I don't even remember what it was. The gathering should have been a warm, joyous experience. But it wasn't. I don't think my wife even came to it.

Lenora: I am sorry about that. They should have done better for you.

Sam: I kind of felt so too. But I've never given it a hell of a lot of thought since.

Lenora: Did you go back to visit afterwards?

Sam: Yes, I went back once or twice. The few people in administration that were still there from my past were very cordial. But not much was going on in my old department. It looked more of a shambles compared to what it was when I was there. I don't know what the hell happened. And the new people in the department seemed uncomfortable in greeting me.

Lenora: It's like your star had set.

Sam: That's a good way to put it.

Lenora: And you know, Sam, you were a tough act to follow.

Sam: Perhaps so, Lenora. Perhaps so.

Note: Sam's tradition lingers on in many Departments of Rehabilitation throughout the country. They are the ones he had set up or those for which he had trained staff over the years. It is ironic that when he was retiring from St.Vincent's, he did not have the opportunity to train successors to his own department.

Consulting for Insurance Companies

Lenora: Can you say something about consulting for insurance companies?

Sam: After I retired, insurance companies did get after me to do work for them.

Lenora: And did you?

Sam: Yes I did.

Lenora: For how long?

Sam: I don't know. At least for the first few years of my retirement.

Lenora: What was that like and how did it fit with you?

Sam: I found it very engaging because it gave me a view of the other side of the fence.

Lenora: What do you mean?

Sam: The insurance companies wanted me as an expert witness mainly in workers' compensation cases. The clients were looking for a big settlement from the insurance company; and the insurance company was always looking for ways to reduce their financial obligation.

Lenora: What was your role in this? What did you do?

Sam: It depended on who was paying my bill.

Lenora: Really? Can you say a little bit more about that?

Sam: Seriously, I had to offer an opinion on how handicapped a worker had become. The worker might be exaggerating pain and limitations, and the insurance company's main interest was reducing the amount of money to settle the case. I had to be aware of both motivations, and be fair in my judgments.

Lenora: How did that work out?

Sam: It required not only thorough physical examinations but also careful observation of the worker's movements and reactions, and documenting my conclusions. When the case went to court, I often had to testify.

Lenora: It kept you busy.

Sam: It wasn't too bad. And I'll tell you the insurance companies paid very well.

Lenora: What a nice part-time activity!

Sam: Yes, it was.

The Last Hurrah

After Sam was widowed, he continued to maintain his home by himself. He was active in the community and enjoyed frequent visits with children and grandchildren. When living alone became too burdensome, he moved in with his daughter and son-in-law and was lovingly cared for. Here is one of our conversations at that time.

Lenora: How do you like the new living arrangements, Sam?

Sam: Delightful. My daughter and son-in-law can't do enough for me. Yet I find the word boredom is in there somewhere. You see, I can`t read well anymore. My balance is poor, and so is my manual dexterity. Physically I am limited.

Lenora: Well, maybe we can do something anyway.

Sam: What do you have in mind?

Lenora: Your speech is fine and your mind is as sharp as ever. Let's collaborate!

Sam: On what?

Lenora: In the past, we often talked about your recording incidents from your medical practice.

Sam: Yes, we did. But I never did anything about it.

Lenora: This is your opportunity!

And that's how this book came to be! For a whole year, Sam recounted incidents to me on the phone. I recorded them, uploaded them into the computer and had them transcribed into text documents. Dr. Sam Sverdlik's Uncommon Stories *is the result of a year of Sam telling me his stories, followed by several months of my compiling and editing the conversations and stories for publication. That was Sam's last year. He was in hospice care at the end.*

Here is part of our last conversation.

Sam: How is it going, Lenora?

Lenora: You mean our project? It's moving along, and I am delighted to be part of this effort.

Sam: Me, too.

Lenora: I don't want to tire you now.

Sam: Yes, I am very tired. I think it's been enough. Yet I am so glad we did all this.

Lenora: I am, too.

Sam: I love you, Lenora.

Lenora: I love you, Sam.

This book is part of Dr. Sam Sverdlik's legacy to the world.

About Dr. Sam Sverdlik

Born in Brooklyn, New York	1916
William and Mary, Williamsburg, VA	1932 -1933
Alfred College, Alfred, NY	1934 -1938
Hahnemann Medical College, Philadelphia, PA	1938 -1942
Married Norma Siegelman	1943
Captain, US Medical Corps, ETO	1943 -1946
MIT Training, Cambridge, MA	1947
Chief Resident, Rusk Rehabilitation Center, NYU-Bellevue Hospital, NY, NY	1947 -1949
Director of Rehabilitation Medicine, St. Vincent's Hospital, New York, NY	1949 -1989
Retired	1989
Widowed	2003
Recorded stories	2013
Died in Fort Myers, FL	2014

Among his many honors are:

1974 American Public Health Association
Award on the 25th anniversary as founder of the first comprehensive rehabilitation unit in a general hospital and Director of Rehabilitation Medicine at the St. Vincent's Hospital and Medical Center, NY, NY.

1988 American Academy of Physical Medicine and Rehabilitation Distinguished Clinician Award

---

Obituary

Samuel Sverdlik passed away peacefully at the age of 97 on the morning of February 2, 2014. Doc Sam was the patriarch of the Sverdlik clan which includes 3 children, 4 grandchildren and 7 great- grandchildren. He savored life every day and always found good everywhere. In lieu of flowers or charitable contributions, the family asks readers to pet a dog, listen to the birds and rejoice in the wonderment of life.

www.ingramcontent.com/pod-product-compliance
Lightning Source LLC
Chambersburg PA
CBHW072309200526

45168CB00014B/1164